KETO LUNCH

Discover 30 Easy to Follow Ketogenic Cookbook Lunch recipes for Your Low-Carb Diet with Gluten-Free and wheat to Maximize your weight loss

STEPHANIE BAKER

AVOCADO CHICKEN BACON SANDWICH

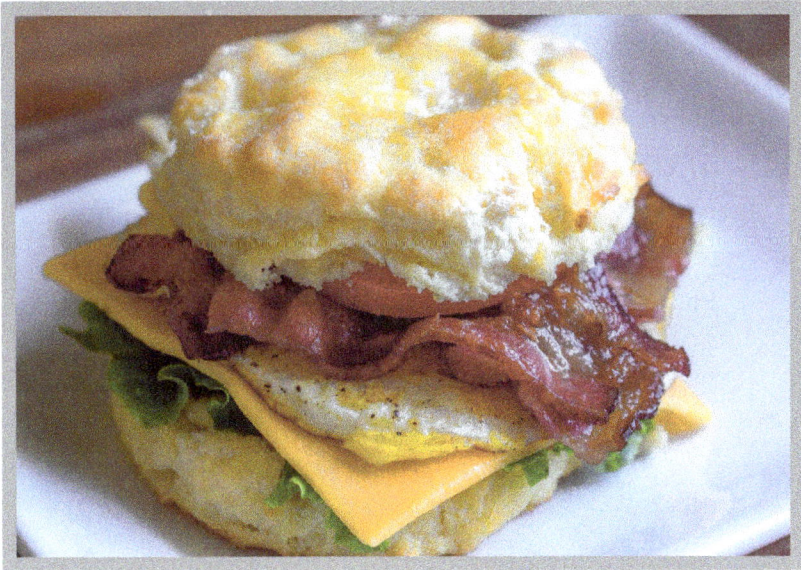

30 min

304 kcal

4 serving

INGREDIENTS

- 1 bread to the cloud
- 2 sliced bacon
- 1 mayonnaise casserole
- 100 g chicken flesh
- 2 cheddar cheese slices
- 1 teaspoon of flying chili goose sauce, sriracha
- 2 tomatoes in wine
- 1/4 advocate

PREPARATION

1. Fry the bacon, and chicken. Add the salt and pepper to the poultry.
2. Brush the cloud sandwich insides with mayo and the hot sriracha sauce.
3. After which put the chicken in the sandwich.
4. Now it's the cheese switch, and the bacon with some tomato slices.
5. Puree the avocado and fill it with cloud bread.

BROCCOLI BACON SALAD

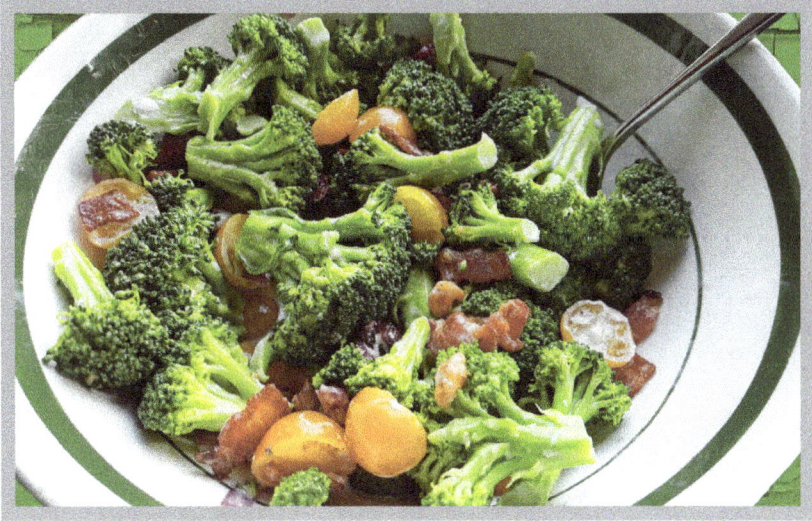

25min

202 kcal

4 serving

INGREDIENTS

- 2 large heads of broccoli
- 200 g sauerkrap
- Shallots: 35 g
- Mayonnaise: 200 g
- 2 tbsp vinegar with white wine
- 3 tbsp stevia oil, or another sweetener
- 1 tinpoon of sesame oil

PREPARATION

1. Briefly cook the bacon until it is moist and crousted.
2. Broccoli cut into pieces.
3. You should cut the shallots to your liking.
4. Then put together the ingredients (mayonnaise, white wine vinegar, sweetener and sesame oil) for dressing.
5. Placed it all into a large bowl of salad.
6. Garnish with crispy little bits of bacon in the salad.

3

LES SALADES DE CESAR

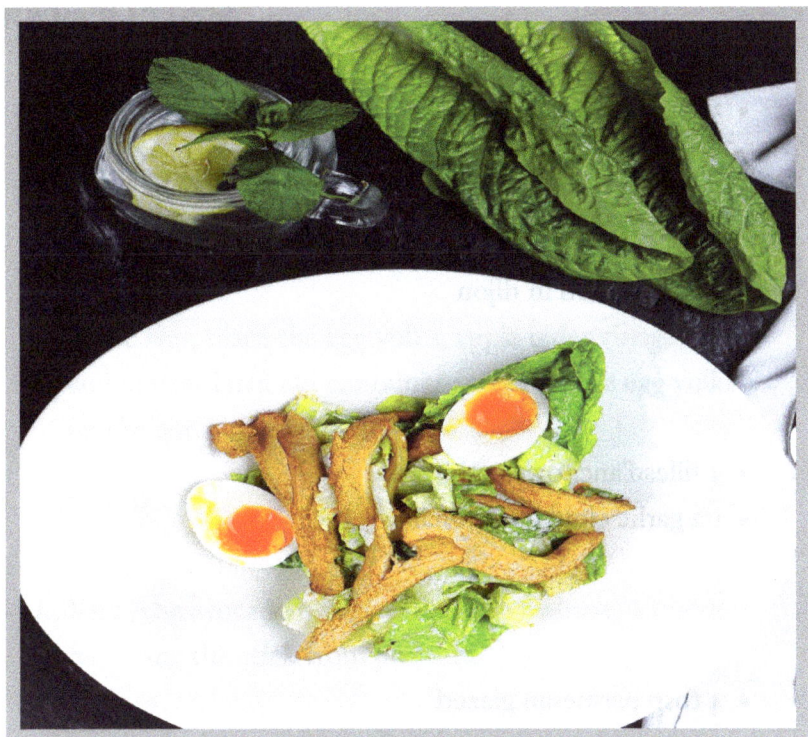

4

CHICKEN PESTO

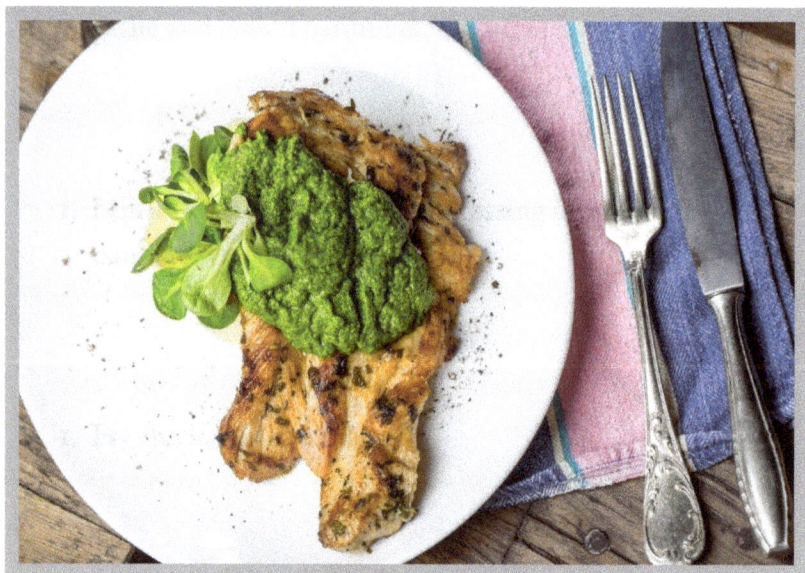

30 min

432 kcal

4 serving

INGREDIENTS

- 4 cups of breadcrumbs

- 1 organic lime / limon zest

- Coconut milk: 360ml

- 1 tassel of new coriander

- 3 or 4 dried chili peppers
- 1 stick of sliced lemongra or 1 tablespoon of dried lemongrace

- A ginger

5

PUREE IN CELERY AND COLIFLOWER

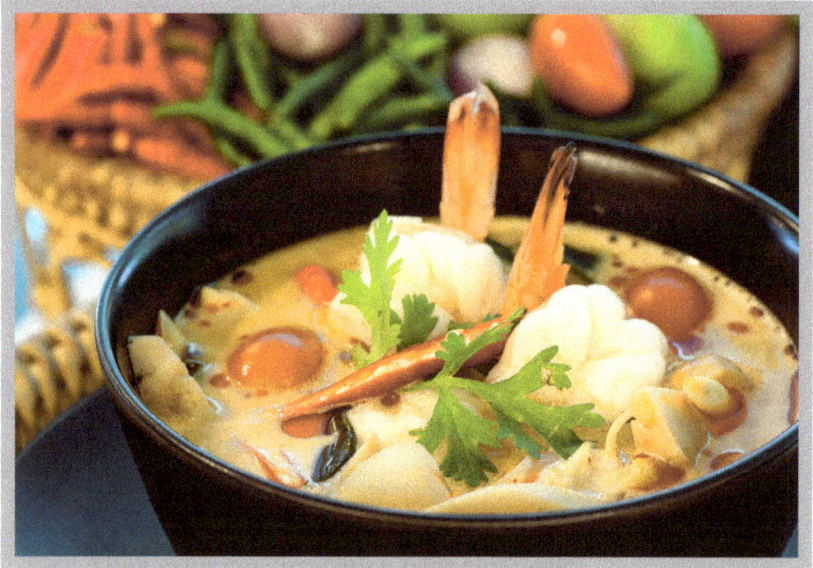

35 min

435kcal

1 serving

INGREDIENTS

- 1 moderate root celery, peeled and cut into cubes

- 1 little head of cauliflower, cut into small florets

- 1/2 cup of salt

- 3 cups of butter

- 2 swiss chard bunches

- 1 cubit butter

- 2 small or large garlic cloves, finely chopped

GRILLED SANDWICH CHEESE

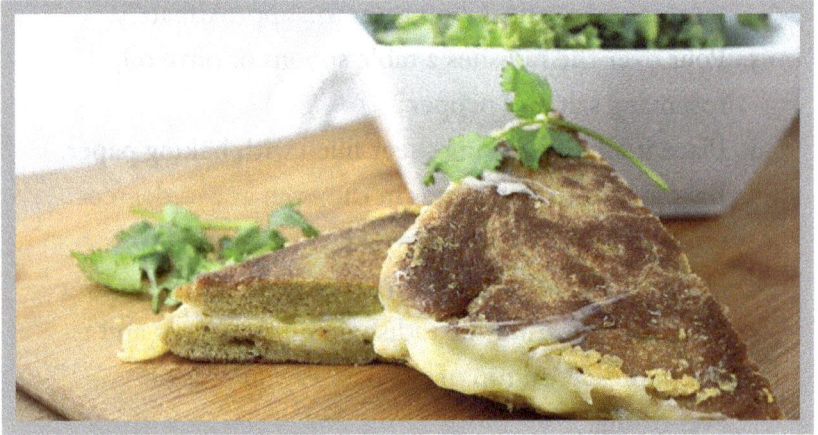

45 min

544kcal

4 serving

INGREDIENTS

- Components in buns

- 2 grand eggs

- 2 spoonfuls of almond flour

- 1 1/2 cubic pound psyllium husk powder

- 1/2 cup of baking powder

- 2 soft butter spoons

- Completes & extras

- 2 units of cheddar cheese

1. Bake the pizza for 10 minutes and remove from the oven. Place the toppings over the pizza and bake for another 8-10 minutes.

1. Remove the pizza from the oven and allow to cool down.

9

SPLENDID JALAPENO POPPERS

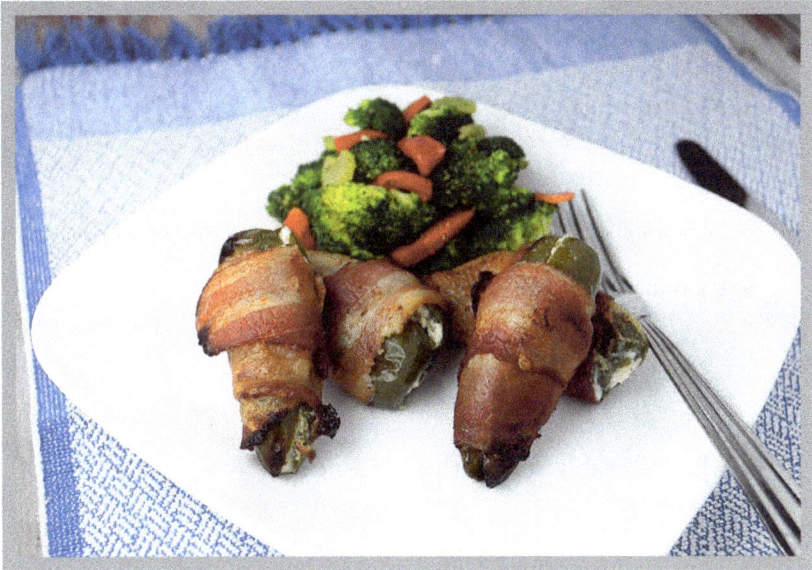

30 min

852 kcal

2 serving

. . .

INGREDIENTS

- 5 units cream cheese

- 1/4 tasse of mozzarella

- 8 medium peppered jalapeno

- 1/4 litre of salt

- 1/4 teaspoon chili pepper

- Ms dash table mix with 1/2 teaspoon

- 8 bacon slices

PREPARATION

1. Oven preheat to 400f. Cut all of the jalapenos in half, and use a knife to remove the peppers' "guts."

1. Mix the cream cheese, mozzarella and your seasoning range in a mug.

1. Pack the mixture of cream cheese in peppers, and place the other half of the pepper on top to close the peppers.

1. In 1 slice of bacon wrap each pepper, starting from the bottom and working up.

1. Bake 20-25 minutes and then fry for 2-3 minutes.

PERSONAL PIZZAS IN PORTOBELLO

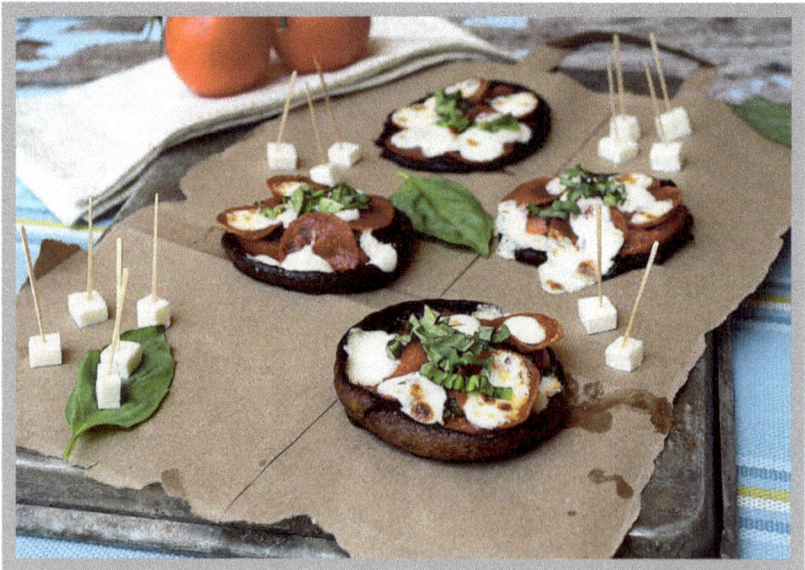

45 min

823 kcal

5 serving

INGREDIENTS

- 4 big caps of champignon portobello

- 1 good tomato wine

- 4 ounces of fresh cheese mozzarella

- 1/4 cup freshly cut basil

- 6 the olive oil spoon

- 20 slices of moist chilies

- Great for salt and pepper

PREPARATION

1. Scrape out the mushroom innards and keep scraping the meat out until the mushroom shell is all you have left.

1. Take the oven to the grill and clean with about 3 table spoons the tops of all the mushrooms. Olive oil, olive oil. Sprinkle with oil and season with salt and pepper.

1. Fry the mushrooms, turn them over and repeat the process for about 4-5 minutes.

1. Cut the tomatoes into thin slices-12-16 slices is enough. Place the tomato on top of the mushrooms, and add the basil.

1. Apply pepperoni to each slice, and sliced mozzarella. Fry for another 2-4 minutes, or until the cheese melts and begins browning.

1. Remove and allow to cool.

GREEN VEGETARIAN COCONUT CURRY

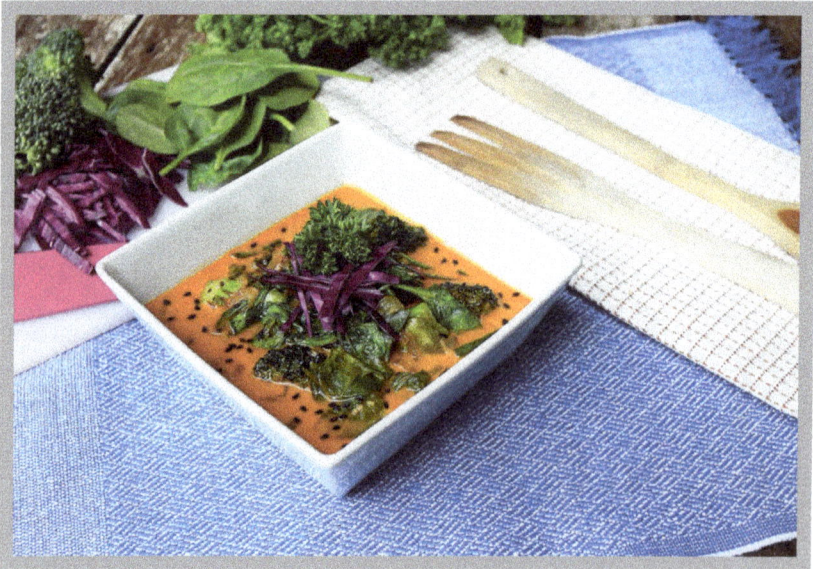

50 min

543 kcal

1 serving

. . .

INGREDIENTS

- 1 cup of broccoli blossoms

- 1 great pack of spinach

- 4 cups of coconut oil

- 1/4 mean onion

- 1 teaspoon of chopped garlic

- 1 teaspoon cut ginger

- 2 cups of fysh sauce

- 2 cups of soy sauce

- 1 twin cubit red curry paste

- 1/2 cup cream for coconut (or milk for coconut)

PREPARATION

1. Split the chopped garlic and the onions. Add 2 dc. Pour coconut oil into a saucepan and heat to medium-high.

1. Attach the onions to the pan after heating, and cook semi-transparently. Then add the garlic to brown in the pan.

1. Switch to medium-low heat and add broccoli to plate. Stir it all up well.

1. When the broccoli is cooked in part, transfer the vegetables to the side of the saucepan and add curry paste. Let it cook within 45-60 seconds.

1. Add spinach to the broccoli and add the coconut cream and the remaining coconut oil once it begins to willow.

1. Add soy sauce, fysh sauce and ginger and mix well. Simmer according to desired thickness for 5-10 minutes.

12

PORK SHIITAKE WITH "FAST KIMCHI" STIR FRY

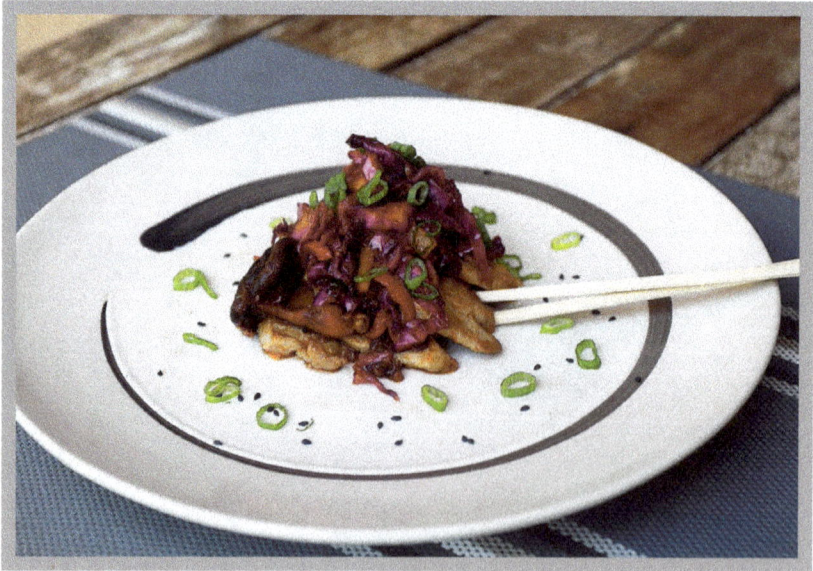

50 min

345 kcal

6 serving

. . .

INGREDIENTS

- kimchi

- 3 cups of purple chopped cabbage

- 3 cups of rice vinegar

- 1 cup of minced garlic

- 2 chopped ginger teaspoons

- 1 1⁄2 cubic lb red boat fish sauce

- 2 teaspoons with red potato flakes

- 1/3 full radish daikon

- 1 giant shallot

- 1 medium red pepper

- 1 twin cubit red curry paste

- 1 1/2 teaspoon soy sauce (or amino acids from the coconut)

- Stir the ingredients into the fry

- 1 pound fresh pork

- 3 lbs of coconut oil

- 3 1⁄2 ounces of champignons shiitake

- 1 giant shallot

- 2 cups of white wine

- 1 spoonful of erythritol now

- 1 1 1⁄2 cubit sesame oil

- Great for salt and pepper

PREPARATION

1. Split the chilli and cabbage into thin strips. Split the radish of a daikon into matches.

1. Combine all the ingredients of "fast kimchi" in a pot, and blend well. Set aside while the pork is being prepared.

1. Cut the pork loin into thin medallions (approx. 1/4 "thick). Apply 1 tablespoon of coconut oil on both sides to cook half the pork before the brown spots emerge.

1. Cut the pork and put it on aside. Then make 1 tbsp to the second batch. Less olive oil.
2. Placed "kimchi" in the saucepan and let the juices boil for 4-5 minutes. Again add pork (with oil) and stir well, allow to cook for another few minutes.

AVOCADO STUFFED WITH EGG SALAD

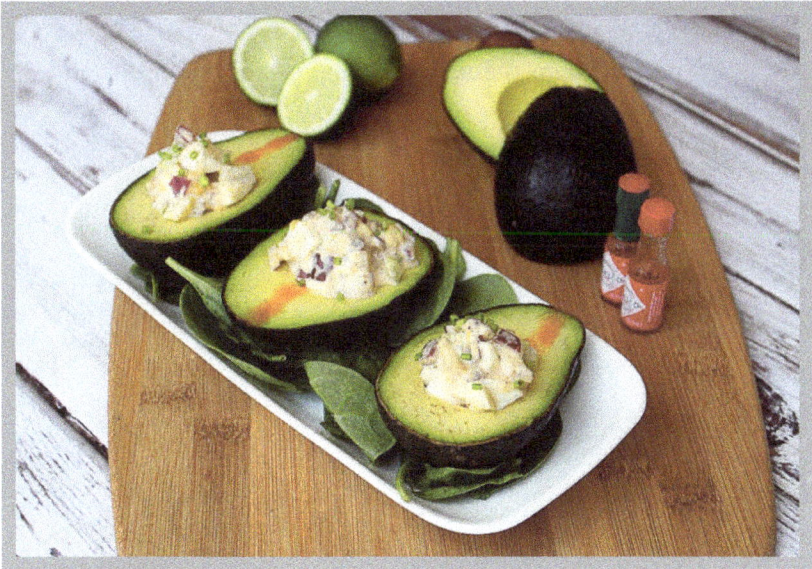

60 min

987 kcal

6 serving

INGREDIENTS

- 6 hard-boiled, big eggs
- 1/3 half red onion
- 3 celery ribs
- 4 cups of mayonnaise
- 2 black mustard teaspoons
- 2 spoonfuls of pure lime juice
- 1 löffel hot sauce
- 1/2 cumin teaspoon
- Great for salt and pepper
- 3 large lawyers

PREPARATION

1. Prepare all ingredients by cutting the eggs, onions and celery into bits.
2. Combine all the ingredients, except avocado, in a dish.
3. Cut the avocado off, and through the seed.
4. Place the avocado egg salad in.

CHEESY WAFFLES WITH THYME

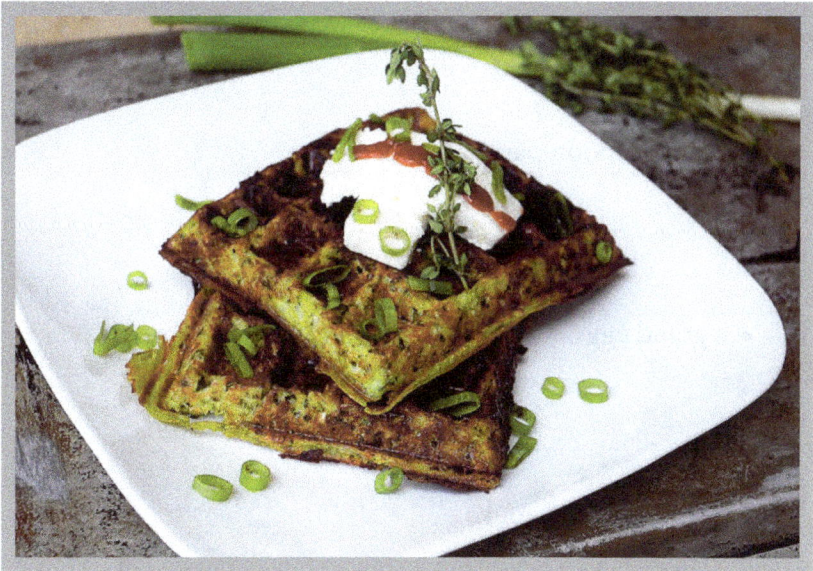

it

70 min

346 kcal

4 serving

INGREDIENTS

- ½ big, mature cauliflower

- 1 cup of fine-cut mozzarella

- 1 cup packed with collard greens

- 1/3 tablespoon parmesan cheese

- 2 grand eggs

- 2 spring-onion sticks

- 1 twin cubit sesame seed

- 1 spoonful of olive oil

- 2 freshly chopped spoonful of thyme

- 1 teaspoon ail dust

- 1/2 teaspoon hot chili pepper

- 1/2 cup of salt

PREPARATION

1. Rice the cauliflower by pulsing the florets in a food processor until it reaches a crumbly texture.

1. Add the chopped vegetables, spring onions, and

thyme and pulse a few more times until all is mixed well.

1. Scoop the mixture into a mixing bowl , add the remaining ingredients and combine well.

1. When dry, pour in the mixture uniformly over a waffle iron frying pan.

1. Cook the mixture until it forms a waffle (as instructed by the manufacturer) then remove.

STUFFED WITH BACON AND BEEF PEPPERS

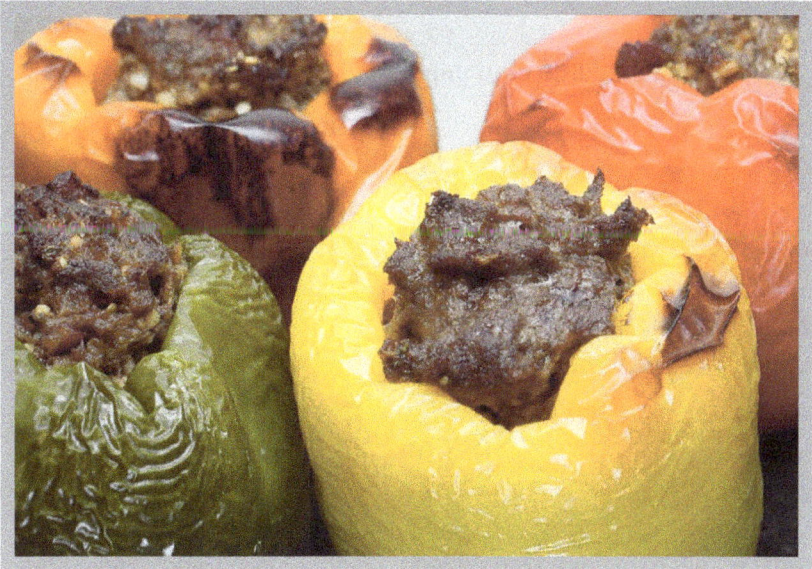

180 min

987 kcal

7 serving

INGREDIENTS

- 1 1/2 lbs of ground beef

- 4 thickly sliced slices of bacon

- 4 small volume chili peppers

- 3 the olive oil spoon

- 1 pound of soy sauce

- 1 cup of minced garlic

- 2 saucer-free ketchup spoons

- 2 oregano teaspoons

- Worcestershire 1 1/2 teaspoon

- 1 löffel hot sauce

- 1 tbsp of liquid smoke

- 1/2 teaspoon hot chili pepper

PREPARATION

1. Place all the meat, butter, and seasonings in a ziploc container. Combine them well before the ingredients are blended together.

1. Marinate this for 3 hours in refrigerator.

1. Have a salted water saucepan boiling on the stove and cut the pepper's center when it comes to boiling.
2. Blanch the peppers, then remove them from the water to dry for 3 minutes.

1. Preheat the oven until 350f

1. Fry some finely chopped bacon, don't absolutely cook it-you just want to par-cook it. When done mix it with the beef.

1. Stuff the peppers with a combination of bacon and beef.

1. Cook the peppers at medium temperature for 50 minutes or until the meat inside.

1. Attach the cheese to the top of the peppers and fry or fry naked to finish with a char.
2. Meatballs with bacon & mozzarella

1. You will see: 155.75 calories, 13.51 g fats, 0.95 g net carbohydrates and 6.98 g protein for each meatball.

16

CHORIZO & CHEDDAR MEATBALLS FOR CHEESE

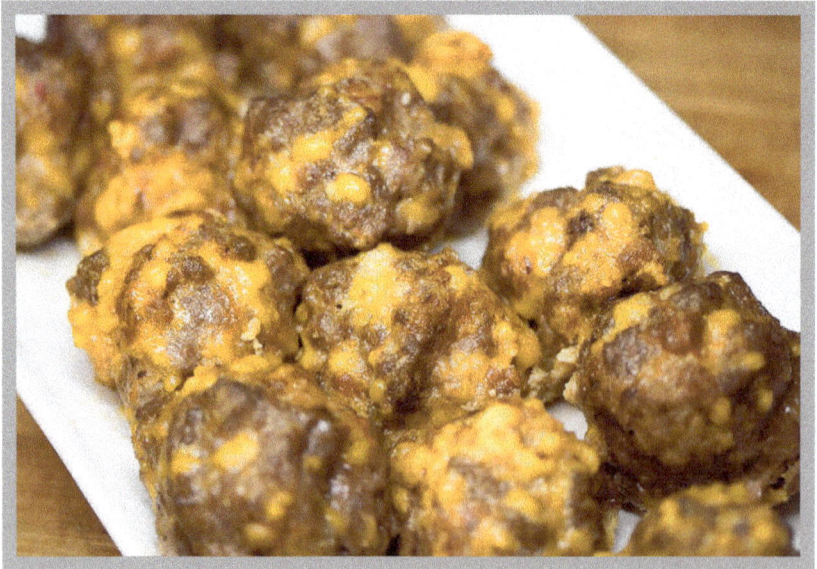

60 min

413 kcal

4 serving

INGREDIENTS

- 1½ lbs of ground beef

- 1 ½ left sausages with chorizo (~ 90 g)

- 1 cup of cheese cheddar

- 1 take some tomato sauce

- Rinds 1/3 cup, cut to bits

- 2 grand eggs

- 1 cumin teaspoon

- 1 teaspoon powdered chili

- 1 kosher salt in teaspoon

PREPARATION

1. Oven preheat to 350f.

1. **Break** the sausage into small bits so the ground beef blends well.

1. Stir in the sausage the ground beef, ground rind, condiments, cheese , and eggs.

1. Blend it all together well before you can shape meatballs.

1. Roll the meatballs out into circles and place them in a baking sheet covered with foil.

1. Bake 30-35 minutes in the oven, or until the meatballs are cooked clean.

1. Pour the tomato sauce and serve over the meatballs.

ITALIAN SAUSAGE MEATBALLS & PEPPERJACK

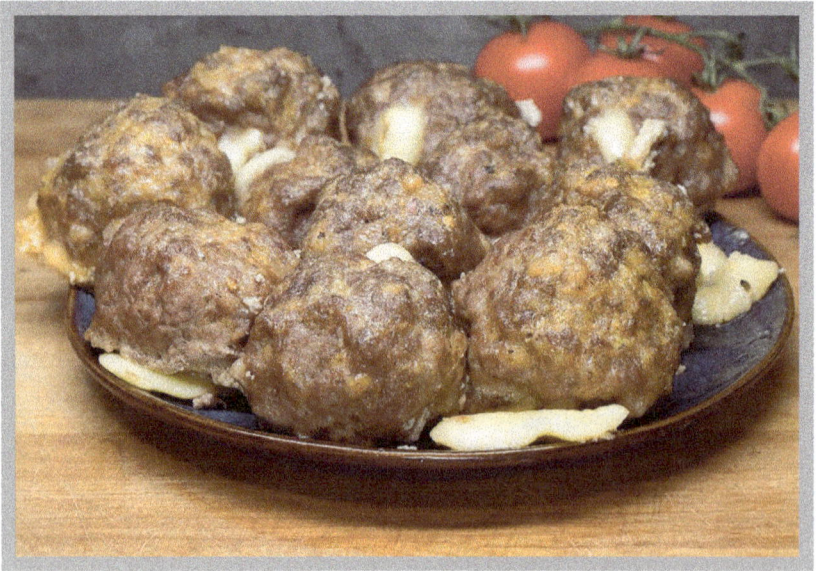

60 min

634 kcal

1 serving

INGREDIENTS

- 1½ lbs of ground beef

- 1 ½ of italian hot sausages left

- 1 cup of sauce with alfredo

- 1/3 cup rinds shredded

- 5 slices of chili cheese

- 2 grand eggs

- 1 oregano teaspoon

- 1 italian seasoning teaspoon

- 1 kosher salt in teaspoon

PREPARATION

1. Oven preheat to 350f.

1. Break the sausage into small bits so the ground beef blends well.

1. In the sausage add the ground beef, ground rind, spices and eggs.

1. Blend it all together well before you can shape meatballs.

1. Take for each meatball 2/3 of the desired amount of meat, and shape it into a semicircle.

1. Place your pepperjack in the middle and top it with some leftover ground beef to seal.

1. Depending on the scale, bak in the oven for 35-45 minutes. The smaller they are, the less cooking time they'll need.

1. Pour over the meatballs, the alfredo sauce and serve.

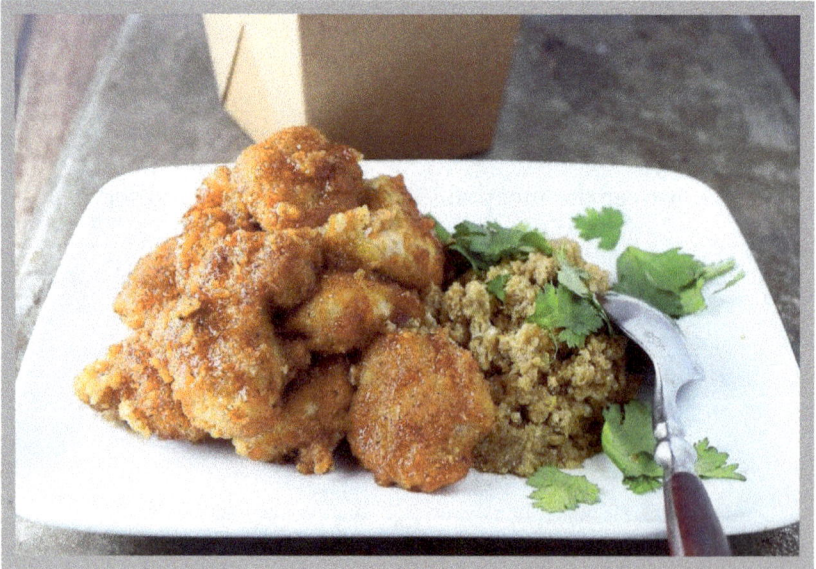

18

SWEET & SOUR LOW CARB CHICKEN

70 min
  453 kcal
  2 serving

INGREDIENTS

- Chicken-chicken:

- 5-6 small boneless chicken branches

- 2 big, beaten eggs

- 1 cup of pork beef, crushed

- 1/2 teaspoon almond flour

- 1/3 tablespoon parmesan cheese

- 2 about tbsp. Petroleum

- 1 pstb. Cocotine oil

- 1 teacup. Salt cosher

- 1 teacup. Black pepper, freshly ground

- Nice sauce with sour colour:

- Erythritol ½ cup

- 1/2 tablespoon rice vinegar

- Four dollars. Reduced ketchup to sugar

- 1 pstb. Soja sauce

- 1 teacup. Ail powder

PREPARATION

1. Main stove

1. Cut the garlic into pieces. In a food processor, combine all the ingredients for the coating and coat the chicken by dipping it in an egg and then in the pork shell crumbs.
2. Cook the chicken over medium heat in batches in a cast iron oven.
3. Reduce the sauce as the chicken cooks in a oven.
4. Brush the sauce into the chicken and blend.

1. Furnace

1. Oven preheat to 325f.

1. Cut off the extra bits, slice the chicken breast.

1. Mash the pork shells and add the flour, salt , pepper and parmesan to the almond.

1. 1 bucket of pounded eggs, 1 tub with a mixture with pork skins.

1. Heat 1 tbsp to the oven. Olive oil and 1 cubic tonsp. Oil extracted from coconut.

1. Sprinkle the chicken cubes in an egg mixture, then mix pork, fry the chicken quickly and put in a baking saucepan, adding more olive oil as needed.
2. Blend the sauce together, and pour over the chicken. Bake 60 minutes, and flip the chicken every 15 minutes.

Remarks

THIS HAS 467 CALORIES, 32 g of fats, 3.9 g of net carbohydrates and 49 g of protein per serving 1.2 pounds.

19

RANCH KING CHICKEN

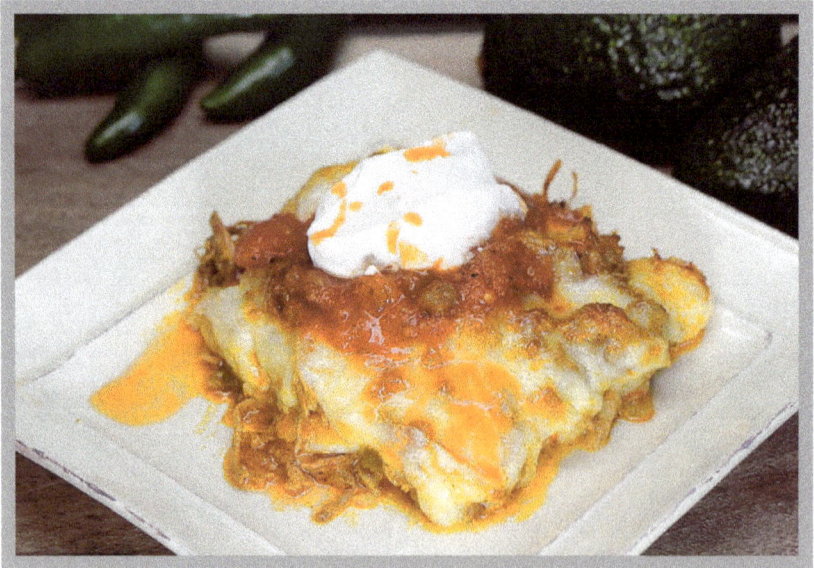

60 min

222 kcal

2 serving

INGREDIENTS

- Cut into bite-sized bits 3 cups of chicken

- 1 cup of breadcrumbs

- 2 liter of butter

- 1/2 little onion, dice

- 1 medium-red, diced potatoes

- 1 twin cubit red chili powder

- 1 cumin teaspoon

- 1 teaspoon ail salt

- 4 ounces of chili peeled orange

- 6 once salsa tomato

- 1⁄2 cup strong crème

- 1/3 tablespoon sour cream

- 16 ounces of jack grated cheese

- 6-7 fabricated tortillas

PREPARATION

1. Cut the chicken into bits of bite size, if you use it raw. Dice paprika and onion.

1. Melt 1 tablespoon butter or coconut oil in a saucepan when using raw chicken, and cook the chicken until ready.

1. Replace, and set aside from the oven. Melt another 1 tablespoon of butter or coconut oil, and cook on medium heat bell pepper and onion for around 5 minutes until tender.
2. Place the spices into the saucepan. Mix well with onions and peppers, and cook, stirring continuously, for about 3 minutes.
3. Remove the broth cup and whisk until all the spice bits are dissolved on the bottom of the saucepan.

1. Add the salsa, chilli and cream and mix well.

1. Cover and simmer for 15 minutes over medium heat, stirring occasionally.

1. Remove 1 1/2 cups of the hot mixture very carefully after 15 minutes, and put them in an emulsion beaker or blender.

1. Blend until thickened. Hold the blender in the bottom of the mug for preventing burns while using an immersion blender.

1. Place the mixed mixture carefully back into the oven.

1. Remove well, and add the yogurt. Combine anything, add meat.

1. In sauce, mix meat and add sauce, tortillas and cheese. Oven preheat to 350 f.

1. Start layering the sauce and meat mixture into a 9x13 baking dish. Simply placed enough to moist the bottom of the plate.

1. Put whole tortillas (don't overlap) in the bottom, then break another tortilla and insert around empty spaces.

1. Layer half of the meat and sauce mixture on the tortillas.

1. Spread half of the cheese uniformly over a mixture of sauce and meat.
2. On the second layer repeat, layer tortillas, then sauce and finish with the remaining cheese mixture. It's headed to furnace!
3. Bake to 350 ° for 30 minutes. Remove from the oven and allow to cool for 10 minutes.
4. Serve, and have fun! Could be surmounted with optional sour cream.

WITH A KICK, LOW CARB CHILI

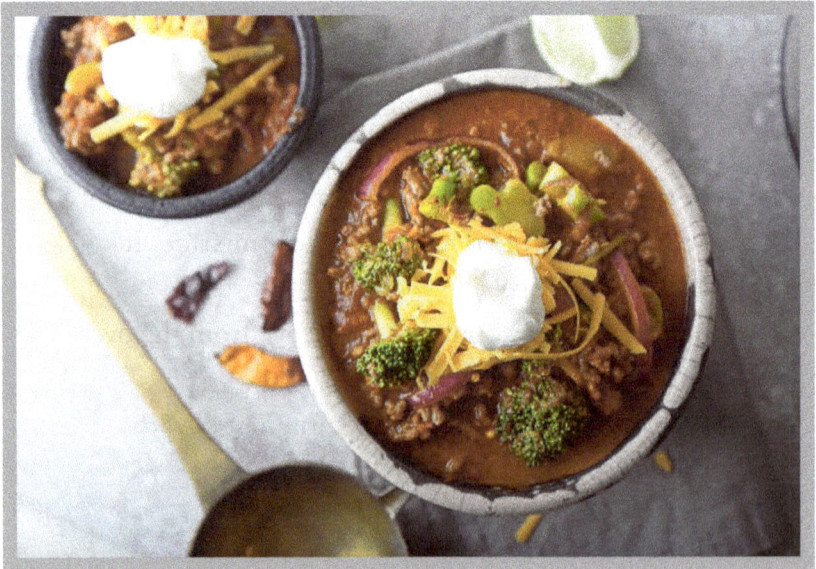

45 min

341 kcal

1 serving

INGREDIENTS

- 1 1/2 lbs of ground beef

- 2 tops of broccoli

- 1 cup of ground beef

- 1 1/2 cans (14.5 ounces each) of jalapeno tomatoes

- 1/2 can green chili (4.5 ounces)

- 1/2 middle-red onion

- 3 medium length stalks of celery

- 1 pound of butter

- 2 cumin teaspoons

- 2 teaspoons of powdered chili

- 1 1/2 garlic teaspoon

- 1 tablespoon of paprika

- 1 teaspoon powdered onion

- 1 italian seasoning teaspoon

PREPARATION

1. Cut the red onions and celery to your liking.

1. Fry the ground beef in a saucepan over high heat in 1 tbsp. Cream. Cream. Garnish with salt and pepper.

1. Start cooking broccoli in a separate saucepan.

1. Once the ground beef begins sizzling, add half of your red onion.

1. Hold your ground beef cooking, and add in the onions so that they can caramelize.

1. Add the celery, remaining onions, green chilli and 1 can of diced tomatoes with jalapeno in your slow cooker.

1. Consume the broccoli and place it in a slow cooker.

1. Place your ground beef and all the fat into the slow cooker.

1. Place your slow cooker on high heat and allow to cook for 20 minutes.

1. Add remaining tomatoes and jalapenos after 20 minutes, and add 1 cup of beef broth.

1. Cover and continue cooking for another 3 hours.

1. Now you can eat it, but i suggest that you leave the top of the slowcooker and let it shrink until less water is in the sauce. It brings the ingredients much more flavor and also makes them more chili-like.

1. Finish with the cheese, or eat it on your own.

21

BACON WRAPPED CORDON BLEU CHICKEN

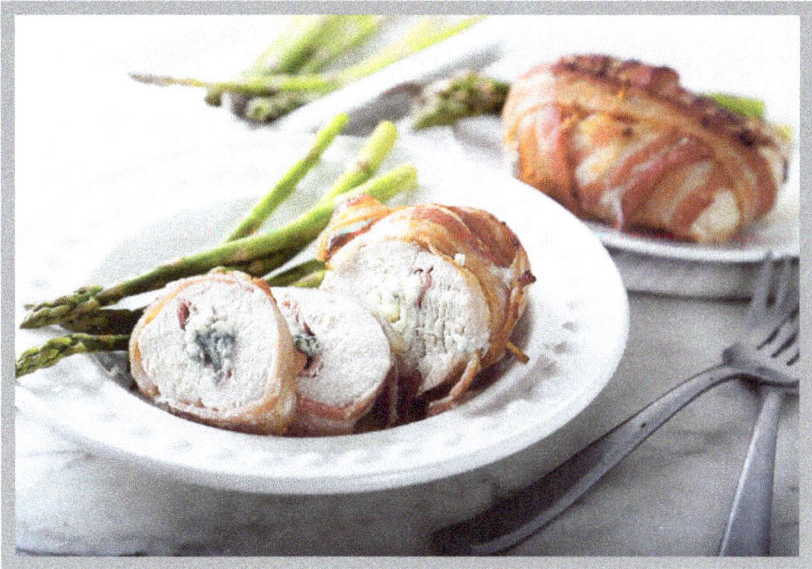

80 min

643 kcal
1 serving

INGREDIENTS

- 2 big, skinless, boneless chicken breasts

- Blue cheese 20ounces

- 4 slices of ham in black forest

- Eight bacon slices

- 12-15 knuckles

PREPARATION

1. The breast meat was cut first. I cut the 2 halves apart and any excess meat off.
2. Cut each part of the breast carefully in half lengthways
3. Place it on top until you launch it, thus cutting it in half. Please ensure all halves remain intact. You don't want to hack through all the way; just enough to put it flat.

1. Place a piece of ham on the breast of the chicken and place the cheese in the middle.

1. Fold 1/3 slice of ham over cheese and fold the remaining 1/3 to close, fold the chicken carefully in half, and cover the ham. Take a piece of bacon and stretch it gently by pulling on both ends. Start from one end and tie the chicken together.

1. Use the second slice of bacon once you have the chicken prepared, and roll it up to the top. If necessary, secure them with toothpicks.

1. Layer the wrapped chicken in an oven-proof pan (i

prefer using cast iron) grated with butter, coconut oil, or bacon-fat.

1. Oven preheat to 3250. Brown bacon over medium heat, on all 4 sides of the pan.

1. Remove the cooker off the pan and put it in the oven. Cook 45 minutes, or until chicken is done. Allow 10 minutes to rest, then serve and enjoy

22

SALMON FILLET WITH PEA AND ALMOND CRUST AND PARSNIP PUREE

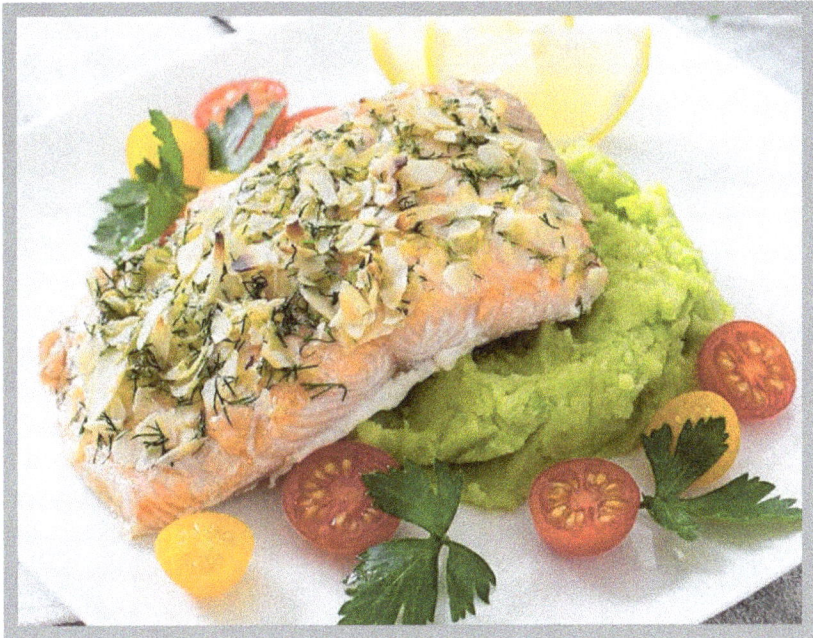

60 min

453 kcal

2 serving

KITCHEN-EQUIPMENT

1 plate, 1 knife,1 casserole ,1 spatula (wood) ,1 casserole,1 potato press,1 wooden spoon,1 table spot, 1 teaspoon.

INGREDIENTS

- 500 g skin salmon filet
- 50 g almonds with flakes

- 2 stalks of dill

- 1 / n lemon

- 1 1 cup of olive oil

- 300 g rough parsnips

- 60 g organic frozen peas

- 50 g craw skinned potatoes

- 50 g milk of cow 3.5 per cent fat

- 50 g sandwiched milk

- 1 preis nutmeg to dry

- 1 roast sea salt (salt fleur)

- 1 black pepper preis

PREPARARTION

1. Select and pat the salmon fillets dry. • heat oil in a

saucepan and fry both sides of the fillets. • wash the
dill, rinse and cut the bark

1. Put the flaked almonds in the empty saucepan and
   combine with your own oil. • pour the salmon fillets
   over the mixture, and season with salt and pepper. •
   cook the fillets over 20 minutes in a preheated oven at
   140-160 ° c.

1. At the same time, peel the parsnips and potatoes and
   cut into small cubes. • cover the vegetables with salted
   water for 10-15 minutes and add the peas just before
   the cooking time is over. • drain the vegetables and let
   them grow in the pot; combine the vegetables with
   milk and whipped cream, and use a potato masher to
   produce it all puree. • spice the pea and puree with
   freshly rubbed nutmeg and salt, then put on two
   plates.

1. Pull the salmon fillets out of the oven with the
   almond crust and put them in the parsnip and pea
   puree.

23

ASIAN SHRIMP CASSEROLE WITH VEGETABLES

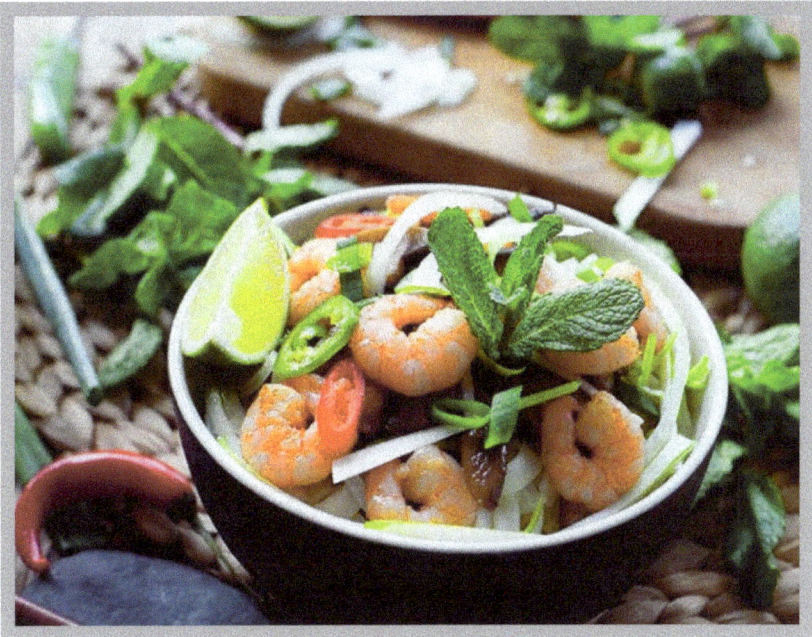

60 min

234 kcal

4 serving

KITCHEN-EQUIPMENT

1 working plate,1 knife,1 cupboard,1 spatula (wood),1 kitchen scale,1 pot, 1 drainer,1 cupboard,1 teaspoon, 1 cupboard,

INGREDIENTS

- 250 g skinless garnelas
- 400 g homemade vegetable broth

- 100 g brown chestnuts

- 40g rice noodles

- 2 onions in the spring

- Tomatoes 1

- 1 lime tail

- 2 garlic nails

- 1/2 pure chilli pepper

- 1 tbsp sauce

- 1 tbsp organic soya sauce

- 1 cup of sesame oil

- 200 ml of warm drinkable water as needed

- 1 tablespoon of sea salt (fleur de sel)

- 1 tablespoon black chili pepper

PREPARATION

1. Rinse and drain the shrimp • clean and cut the mushrooms into slices • clean the spring onions and cut them into rings • wash the tomatoes and cut them into small cubes • peel the garlic and cut into thin slices • cut the chili peppers into thin rings.

1. In a saucepan heat the vegetable broth, remove the casserole from heat and cook the rice noodles in it. • in a saucepan , heat the sesame oil and cook the prawns quickly with garlic. • pour in the mushrooms, chilies and tomatoes and fry them.

1. Break the lime, and suck the juice out. • blend 200 ml of hot water with a fish sauce, soy sauce and a little lime juice, then add to the tub. • add the spring onions and use salt and pepper to season everything. • swirl in the rice noodles, then blend properly.
2. Add a little vegetable stock if necessary, and then season with salt, pepper and lime juice again. • put the asian pan into two bowls with shrimp and vegetables and serve.

1. Hint: of course low-carbohydrate noodles from the konjac root also fit perfectly in the recipe and you can reduce the carbohydrate count even more.

24

BEETROOT SALAD WITH FETA AND ORANGE

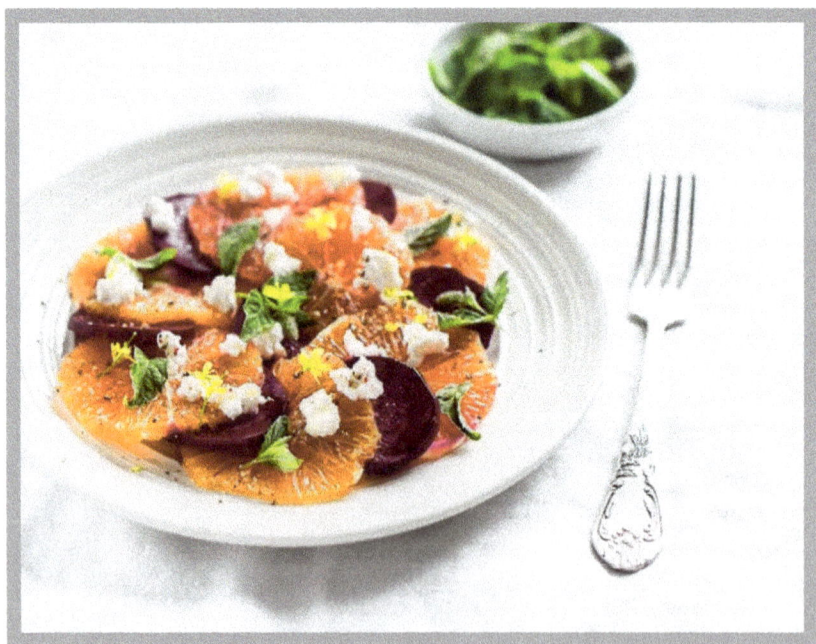

50 min

305 kcal

2 serving

KITCHEN-EQUIPMENT

1 working plate ,one knife, one kitchen scale, one lemon squeezer, one teaspoon

INGREDIENTS

- 200 g crude beetroot

- Orange: 70 g

- Feta: 30 g

- 1 mince-stalk

- 1/2 lime newly squeezed

- Chili flakes 1/2 tsp, as needed

- 1 tablespoon of salt from the sea (fleur de sel)

- 1 tablespoon black chili pepper

PREPARATION

1. Scrape the beetroot-preferably with protective gloves-
   and cut into slices • generously cut the orange so that
   the skin is cut off, then cut into slices • instead put
   the orange and beetroot slices on a plate.
2. Rinse the mint. Then you pluck your seeds. • crumble
   the feta into your palm and spill over slices of orange
   and beetroot.

25

COLORFUL SPINACH SALAD, MANGO, ALMONDS AND DRESSING

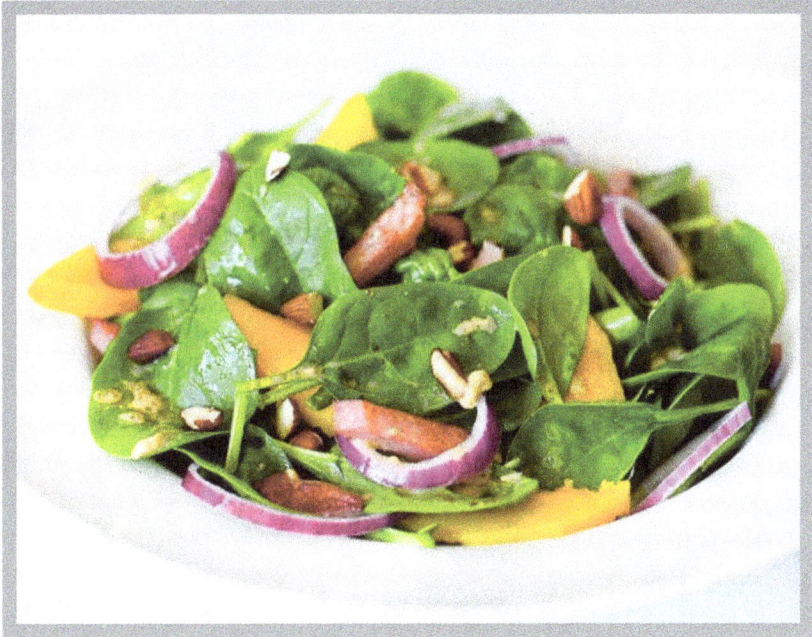

40 min

443 kcal

2 serving

KITCHEN-EQUIPMENT

1 ipad, 1 knife, 1 salad bowl, 1 salad spinner,1 kitchen scale,1 cupboard,1 teaspoon

INGREDIENTS

- 200 g new baby spinach

- Mango 100 g

- 150 g new red potatoes

- 30 g mandarins

- 30 g red ointment

- 150 g treat

- 50 ml potable water
- 1 raw lime, freshly pressed

- 1 tbsp cider apple vinegar

- 1 tsp artichoke syrup

- 2 coriander stems, new,

- 1 peppered chili (raw)
- 1 a garlic clove

- 1 tablespoon of salt from the sea (fleur de sel)

- 1 tablespoon black chili pepper

PREPARATION

1. For the dressing, cut the peeled mango pulp into cubes. • wash and dry the cilantro, then pluck the leaves and chop. • garlic peel. • halve the pepper chilli and cut seeds.

2. Within a blender jar place the mango, sugar, lime juice, apple cider vinegar, maple syrup, chilli and garlic and puree all with the hand blender. • add salt and pepper to the dressing and stir in chopped coriander leaves.

3. Rinse the leaves of spinach for the salad, and dry them in a salad spinner. • cut the too long stalks of the spinach leaves and take the too large leaves.

4. Peel the onion and cut it into rings • cut the peeled mango into strips • finely chop the almonds • in a salad bowl, put the spinach, mango, bell pepper, almonds and onion and drizzle with the dressing, mix all and place on two plates.

26

CHICKEN BREAST WITH OLIVES, ONIONS AND CHARD

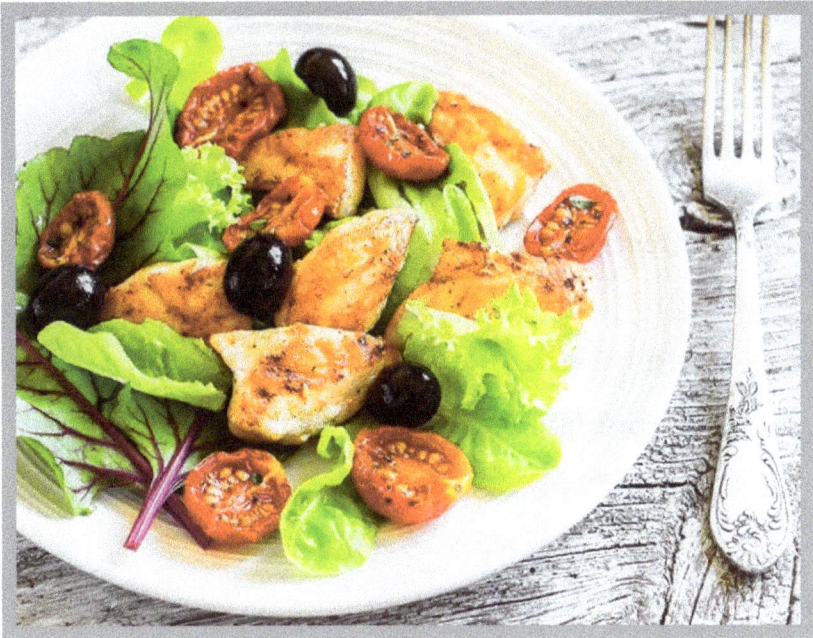

60 min

340 kcal

2 serving

KITCHEN-EQUIPMENT

1 working pan,1 knife,1 kitchen scale,1 casserole,1 grill tongs,
1 salad spinner,1 cupboard,1 teaspoon.

INGREDIENTS

- 250 g breast chicken

- Chard 50 g

- 30 g romanesque salad

- 50 g coarse black olives

- 100 g loved tomatoes

- 2 spoonfuls of olive oil

- 1 tablespoon of salt from the sea (fleur de sel)

- 1 tablespoon black chili pepper

PREPARATION

1. Rinse the leaves of chard and romana lettuce, and dry them in a spinner of salad. • cut the leaves into bits of lettuce and place them on a platter. • wash tomatoes, and halve them. • remove the olives;
2. Rinse the breast filet for the chicken, pat it dry and cut into slices. • heat the oil in the saucepan and cook the meat pieces until golden brown. Placed the tomatoes in the saucepan a little before the finish of the cooking process.

1. Season with salt and pepper and apply warm to the salad. • top with olives and serve.

27

COURGETTE BAKE WITH MOZZARELLA AND SWEET POTATOES

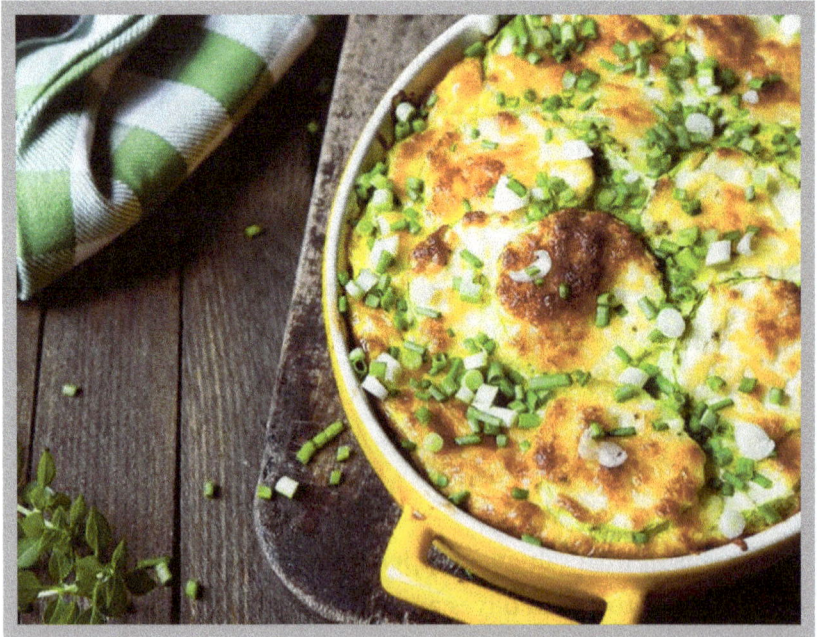

120 min

453 kcal
1 serving

KITCHEN EQUIPMENT

1 work plate, 1 knife,1 kitchen scale,1 kettle,1 wooden spoon,1 measuring cup, 1 baking platter,1 grater,1 table spoon,1 teaspoon.

INGREDIENTS

- 300 grams of courgettes

- 100 g / n sweet potatoes

- 1 springtime onion / s

- 2 knob cloves

- 4 sticks of petersil

- 150 g mozzarella rubbed

- 200 ml of cow's milk 1.5% fat

- 50 ml of whipped cream-30%

- 2 cups of butter

- Type 630 10 g spelled flour

- 1 pinch of dried muscat
- 1 tablespoon of salt from the sea (fleur de sel)

- 1 tablespoon black chili pepper

- Drinking water according to need

PREPARATION

1. Wash the zucchini and rinse, and cut the ends off. •
   cut the courgettes uniformly into approximately 5 mm
   thick slices. • cut and cut the sweet potato into thin
   slices.

1. Scrape and chop the garlic • wash the parsley and dry
   it, then pluck and chop the leaves • clean the onions
   from the spring and cut into rings.

1. Melt the butter in a saucepan and stir with a whisk in
   the seasoned flour. • add the milk and stir well so no
   lumps are produced.

1. Stir in the milk and season with freshly grated
   nutmeg, salt and pepper. • stir in a little more water, if
   the sauce gets too thick. In the sauce put the garlic
   and parsley, and stir. • add the zucchini and the sweet
   potato and boil with the lid closed for a short time.
2. Get it all fireproof, then sprinkle it with mozzarella. •
   cook the whole thing over 30-40 minutes in a
   preheated oven at 180 ° c.
3. After 30 minutes , take the casserole out and test that

the vegetables are cooked with a fork. Otherwise keep cooking on in the oven. • remove the saucepan from the oven, sprinkle with the onion rings and eat.

CAULIFLOWER HASH WITH FRIED EGG BROWNS

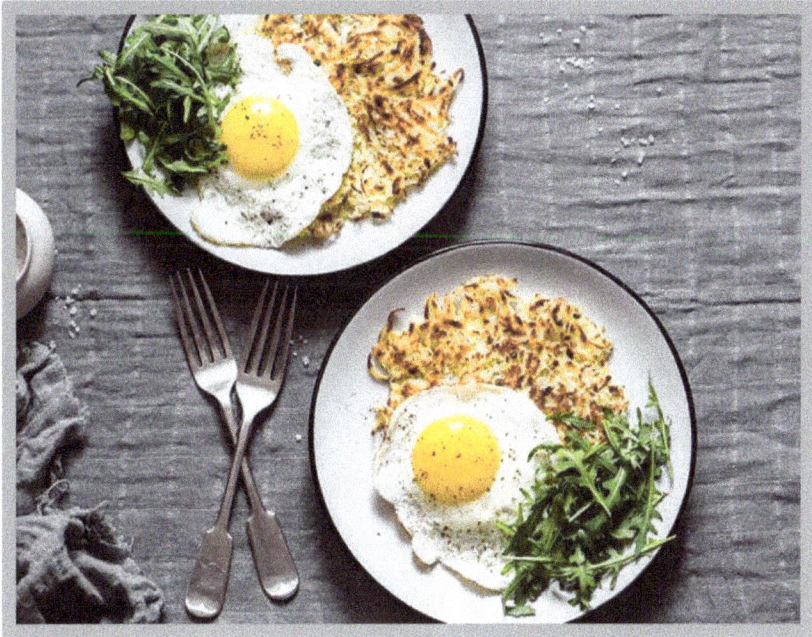

40 min

289 kcal

2 serving

KITCHEN-EQUIPMENT

1 working plate, 1 knife, 1 casserole, 1 spatula, 1 pot, 1 grater, 1 kitchen scale, 1 cubicle, 1 teaspoon.

INGREDIENTS

For certain hash browns

- Cauliflower 300 g, rubberised

- 80 g, rubbed potato

- 1 egg, dimensions m.

- Muskat

- 1 1 cup of olive oil

- For those fried eggs
- 2 chickens, weigh m.

- 2 tspoon butter

- Olive oil 1 tsp.

- Furthermore,

- 30 g rabbit

- Seafood

- Pepper

PREPARATION

1. Mix the egg in a bowl with the rubbed potatoes and cauliflower for the röstis and season the mixture with salt , pepper and freshly grated nutmeg. • heat the oil in a pan and add parts of the roasted mixture (depending on the pan size).

1. Place the spatula fairly flat on the rösti and turn them over after a few minutes. • at the other hand, cook the hash browns, take out the next part and prepare them in the same way.

1. In a second pan , heat up the butter and oil. • beat the eggs gently, and add them.
2. While wash the leaves of the rocket and shake it out, then add a serving to each dish. • add brown hash cauliflower and fried eggs, then serve.

1. hint: the rösti can be kept warm in the oven at 50 ° c for larger portions before all the rösti are fried.

29

LOW CARBONATED SALMON- AND AVOCADO BREAD

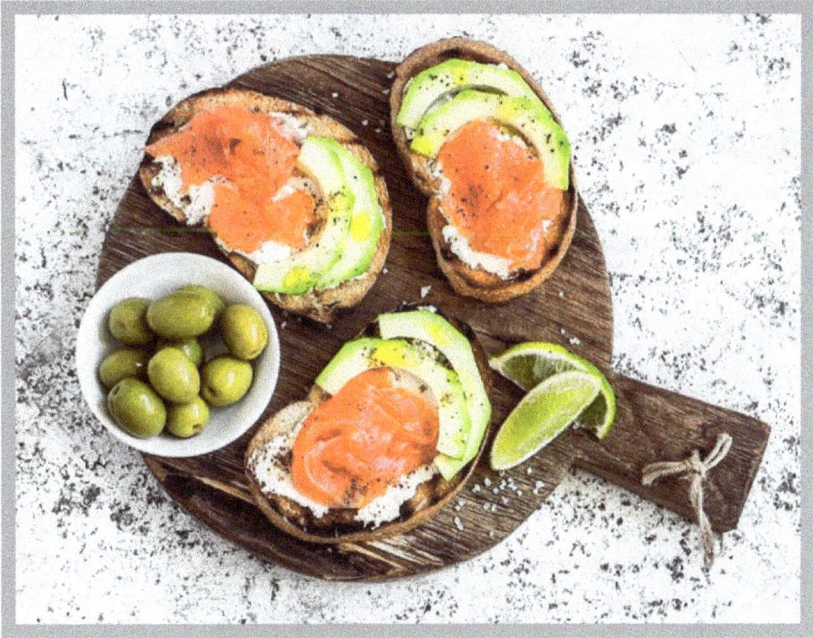

10 min

804 kcal

1 serving

KITCHEN-EQUIPMENT

1 working board, 1 knife, 1 grill tongs, 1 grill or 1 toaster, 1 spoonful.

INGRDIENTS

- 3 low carbohydrate slices of bread from our cookbook

- 70 g smoked wild salmon

- 60 grams of black olives

- 1/2 lawyer

- 1 lime tail

- Butter 20 g

- 1 1 cup of olive oil

- Water salt (salt fleur)

- Pepper

PREPARATION

1. Cut the avocado in half and remove the kernel, strip the pulp from the skin and cut into slices. • cut the lime, squeeze the juice out and drizzle over the slices of the avocado so that the pulp stays green and does not turn brown.
2. Toast low-carb slices of bread in a toaster or on a hot grill pan. • place the bread on the plate, brown it with butter and add the avocado and wild salmon on top. • spray with olive oil on the avocado and sauté with salt and pepper olives.

30

HOMEMADE MEATBALLED TOMATO SOUP

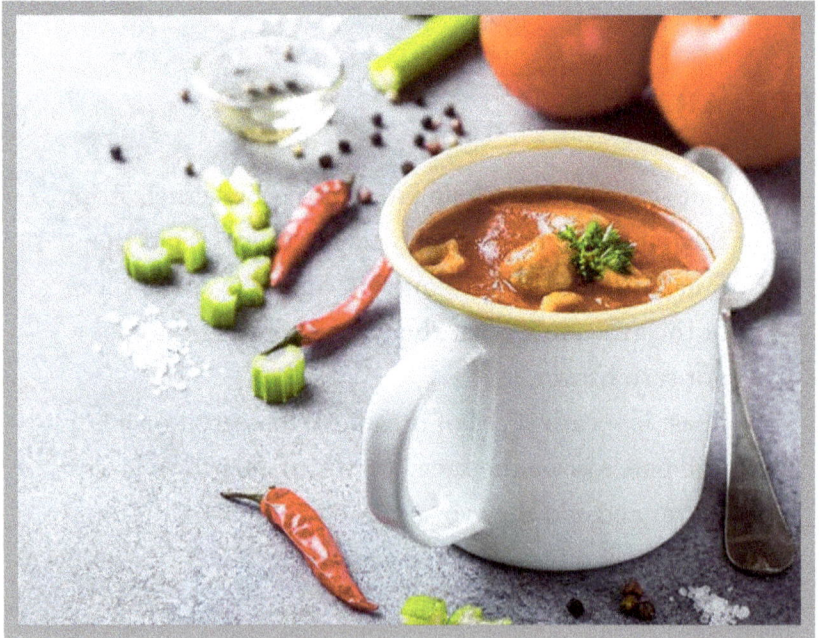

60 min

608 kcal

6 serving

KITCHEN-EQUIPMENT

1 tablet, 1 knife, 1 pot, 1 wooden spoon, 1 cup, 1 kitchen scale, 1 spoon.

INGREDIENTS

- Passata 400 ml
- 400 g natural preservative tomatoes
- 2 shoals
- 2 celery sticks (raw celery), raw,
- 2 knuckles
- 1 peppered chili (raw)
- 400 g boiled beef
- 1 scale of an egg m.
- 1 table litre of yogurt in greek style
- 4 petersil stalks
- 2 from new thyme stems
- 2 mezzanines of olive oil
- 1 tsp of salt (salt flower)
- 1 tablespoon black chili pepper
- Pasta 150 g – chickpeas

PREPARATION

1. Clean and cut into pieces fresh tomatoes and remove the base. • cut the shallots, and finely dice them. • clean, wash, and thinly cut celery stalks. Peel the garlic, and slice it finely. Cut the chilli pepper, halve, core and chop.

1. In a large saucepan heat up the olive oil and sauté the shallots with garlic. • stir in celery and tomatoes, and fire. • bring chilli and passata to a boil. • cover medium heat tomato soup and allow to simmer.

1. Wash the herbs for the meatballs and shake them dry, then pick the leaves, and finely chop them. • in a pot, beat the egg and add the minced beef, yoghurt and herbs. • mix in a little salt and pepper and blend well.

1. Shape tiny balls with wet hands out of the mixture of minced meat. • in a saucepan, add olive oil and cook the meatballs until golden brown. • then remove the meatballs from the saucepan and set aside.

1. Prepare low-carbohydrate pasta as instructed, drain
   and allow to drain in a colander. • re-sawn the tomato
   soup. • puree the soup with a hand blender, if you
   like it.

www.ingramcontent.com/pod-product-compliance
Lightning Source LLC
Chambersburg PA
CBHW050738030426
42336CB00012B/1623